Nothing is so
firmly believed
as that which
we least know.

-Michel de
Montaigne

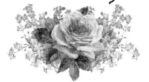

MONDAY_____

_____

_____

TUESDAY_____

_____

_____

WEDNESDAY_____

_____

_____

THURSDAY_____

_____

_____

FRIDAY_____

_____

_____

SATURDAY_____ **SUNDAY**_____

_____

_____

GOALS

_____

_____

_____

_____

NOTES

_____

_____

_____

_____

_____

_____

_____

_____

_____

_____

_____

_____

_____

_____

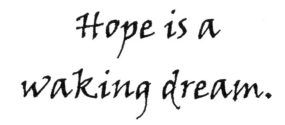

Hope is a
waking dream.

-Aristotle

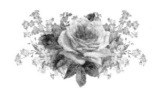

MONDAY_____

_____

_____

_____

TUESDAY_____

_____

_____

_____

WEDNESDAY_____

_____

_____

THURSDAY_____

_____

_____

_____

FRIDAY_____

_____

_____

_____

SATURDAY_____   **SUNDAY**_____

_____

_____

GOALS

_____

_____

_____

_____

_____

NOTES

_____

_____

_____

_____

_____

_____

_____

_____

_____

_____

_____

_____

_____

The wisest men
follow their own
direction.

-Euripides

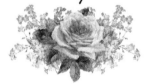

MONDAY_____

_____

_____

_____

TUESDAY_____

_____

_____

_____

WEDNESDAY_____

_____

_____

THURSDAY_____

_____

_____

_____

FRIDAY_____

_____

_____

_____

SATURDAY_____ SUNDAY_____

_____

_____

GOALS

_____

_____

_____

_____

_____

NOTES

_____

_____

_____

_____

_____

_____

_____

_____

_____

_____

_____

_____

_____

_____

_____

_____

You can only
fight the way
you practice.

-Miyamoto
Musashi

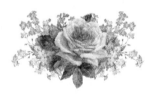

MONDAY_____

_____

_____

_____

TUESDAY_____

_____

_____

_____

WEDNESDAY_____

_____

_____

THURSDAY_____

_____

_____

_____

FRIDAY_____

_____

_____

_____

SATURDAY_____ **SUNDAY**_____

_____

_____

_____

GOALS

NOTES

An ounce of
action is worth a
ton of theory.

-Friedrich Engels

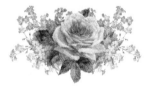

MONDAY_____

_____

_____

TUESDAY_____

_____

_____

WEDNESDAY_____

_____

_____

THURSDAY_____

_____

_____

_____

FRIDAY_____

_____

_____

_____

SATURDAY_____   **SUNDAY**_____

_____

_____

GOALS

_____

_____

_____

_____

_____

NOTES

_____

_____

_____

_____

_____

_____

_____

_____

_____

_____

We are what we
repeatedly do.
Excellence,
then, is not an
act, but a habit.

-Aristotle

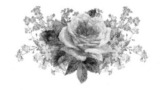

MONDAY_____

TUESDAY_____

WEDNESDAY_____

THURSDAY_____

FRIDAY_____

SATURDAY_____ **SUNDAY**_____

GOALS

NOTES

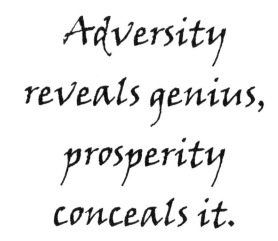

Adversity
reveals genius,
prosperity
conceals it.

~Horace

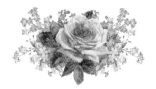

MONDAY_____

_____

_____

TUESDAY_____

_____

_____

WEDNESDAY_____

_____

_____

THURSDAY_____

_____

_____

FRIDAY_____

_____

_____

SATURDAY_____   SUNDAY_____

_____

_____

GOALS

_____

_____

_____

_____

_____

NOTES

_____

_____

_____

_____

_____

_____

_____

_____

_____

_____

_____

_____

_____

_____

Life grants
nothing to us
mortals without
hard work..

-Horace

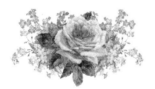

MONDAY＿＿＿＿＿

GOALS

TUESDAY＿＿＿＿＿

WEDNESDAY＿＿＿＿＿

NOTES

THURSDAY＿＿＿＿＿

FRIDAY＿＿＿＿＿

SATURDAY＿＿＿＿＿　　**SUNDAY**＿＿＿＿＿

Life will only
change when
you become more
committed to
your dreams
than your
comfort zone.

-Unknown

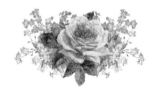

MONDAY_____

_____

_____

_____

TUESDAY_____

_____

_____

_____

WEDNESDAY_____

_____

_____

_____

THURSDAY_____

_____

_____

_____

FRIDAY_____

_____

_____

_____

SATURDAY_____   **SUNDAY**_____

_____

_____

GOALS

_____

_____

_____

_____

_____

_____

NOTES

_____

_____

_____

_____

_____

_____

_____

_____

_____

_____

_____

_____

_____

Do not judge,
and you will
never be
mistaken.

-Jean Jacques
Rousseau

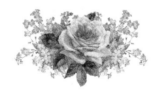

MONDAY_____

TUESDAY_____

WEDNESDAY_____

THURSDAY_____

FRIDAY_____

SATURDAY_____   SUNDAY_____

GOALS

NOTES

And say my
glory was I had
such friends.

-W. B. Yeats

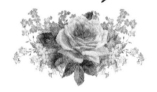

MONDAY_____

_____

_____

_____

TUESDAY_____

_____

_____

_____

WEDNESDAY_____

_____

_____

_____

THURSDAY_____

_____

_____

_____

FRIDAY_____

_____

_____

_____

SATURDAY_____   **SUNDAY**_____

_____

_____

GOALS

_____

_____

_____

_____

_____

_____

NOTES

_____

_____

_____

_____

_____

_____

_____

_____

_____

_____

_____

_____

_____

Plunge boldly into
the thick of life,
and seize it where
you will, it is
always interesting.

-Johann Wolfgang
von Goethe

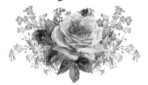

MONDAY_____

GOALS

TUESDAY_____

WEDNESDAY_____

NOTES

THURSDAY_____

FRIDAY_____

SATURDAY_____ **SUNDAY**_____

The aim of art is
to represent not
the outward
appearance of
things, but
their inward
significance.

-Aristotle

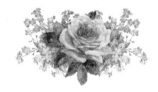

MONDAY_____

TUESDAY_____

WEDNESDAY_____

THURSDAY_____

FRIDAY_____

SATURDAY_____   SUNDAY_____

GOALS

NOTES

You have power
over your mind —
not outside
events. Realize
this, and you
will find
strength.

-Marcus Aurelius

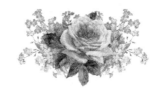

MONDAY_____

_____

_____

TUESDAY_____

_____

_____

WEDNESDAY_____

_____

THURSDAY_____

_____

_____

FRIDAY_____

_____

_____

SATURDAY_____   SUNDAY_____

_____

_____

GOALS

_____
_____
_____
_____
_____

NOTES

_____
_____
_____
_____
_____
_____
_____
_____
_____
_____
_____
_____
_____

You can't wait
for inspiration.
You have to go
after it with
a club.

-Jack London

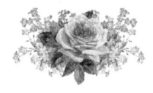

MONDAY_____

_____

_____

_____

TUESDAY_____

_____

_____

_____

WEDNESDAY_____

_____

_____

_____

THURSDAY_____

_____

_____

_____

FRIDAY_____

_____

_____

_____

SATURDAY_____ **SUNDAY**_____

_____

_____

GOALS

_____

_____

_____

_____

_____

NOTES

_____

_____

_____

_____

_____

_____

_____

_____

_____

_____

_____

_____

_____

Man is never perfect, nor contented.

-Jules Verne

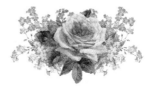

MONDAY_____

_____

_____

_____

TUESDAY_____

_____

_____

_____

WEDNESDAY_____

_____

_____

_____

THURSDAY_____

_____

_____

_____

FRIDAY_____

_____

_____

_____

SATURDAY_____ **SUNDAY**_____

_____

_____

_____

GOALS

_____

_____

_____

_____

_____

_____

NOTES

_____

_____

_____

_____

_____

_____

_____

_____

_____

_____

_____

_____

_____

_____

If you care
enough for a
result, you will
most certainly
attain it.

-William James

MONDAY_____

_____

_____

_____

TUESDAY_____

_____

_____

_____

WEDNESDAY_____

_____

_____

_____

THURSDAY_____

_____

_____

_____

FRIDAY_____

_____

_____

_____

SATURDAY_____   **SUNDAY**_____

_____

_____

_____

GOALS

_____

_____

_____

_____

_____

_____

NOTES

_____

_____

_____

_____

_____

_____

_____

_____

_____

_____

_____

_____

_____

The proper function
of man is to live,
not to exist. I shall
not waste my days
in trying to prolong
them. I shall
use my time.

-Jack London

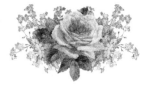

MONDAY_____
_____
_____
_____

TUESDAY_____
_____
_____
_____

WEDNESDAY_____
_____
_____
_____

THURSDAY_____
_____
_____
_____

FRIDAY_____
_____
_____
_____

SATURDAY_____   **SUNDAY**_____
_____
_____

GOALS

_____
_____
_____
_____
_____
_____

NOTES

_____
_____
_____
_____
_____
_____
_____
_____
_____
_____
_____
_____
_____

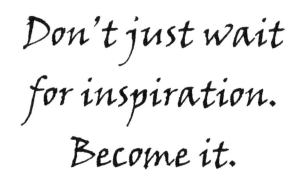

Don't just wait
for inspiration.
Become it.

-Unknown

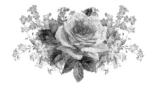

MONDAY_____

_____
_____
_____

TUESDAY_____

_____
_____
_____

WEDNESDAY_____

_____
_____

THURSDAY_____

_____
_____
_____

FRIDAY_____

_____
_____

SATURDAY_____   SUNDAY_____

_____
_____

GOALS

_____
_____
_____
_____
_____
_____

NOTES

_____
_____
_____
_____
_____
_____
_____
_____
_____
_____
_____
_____
_____
_____
_____

You are free,
and that is why
you are lost.

-Franz Kafka

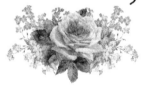

MONDAY_____

TUESDAY_____

WEDNESDAY_____

THURSDAY_____

FRIDAY_____

SATURDAY_____ **SUNDAY**_____

GOALS

NOTES

Just as a candle
cannot burn
without fire,
men cannot live
without a
spiritual life.

-Buddha

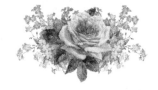

MONDAY_____

TUESDAY_____

WEDNESDAY_____

THURSDAY_____

FRIDAY_____

SATURDAY_____　　**SUNDAY**_____

GOALS

NOTES

Faith is to believe what you do not yet see; the reward for this faith is to see what you believe.

-Augustine of Hippo

MONDAY_____

GOALS

TUESDAY_____

WEDNESDAY_____

NOTES

THURSDAY_____

FRIDAY_____

SATURDAY_____   **SUNDAY**_____

It is not in the
stars to hold our
destiny but in
ourselves.

-William
Shakespeare

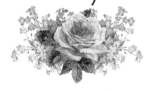

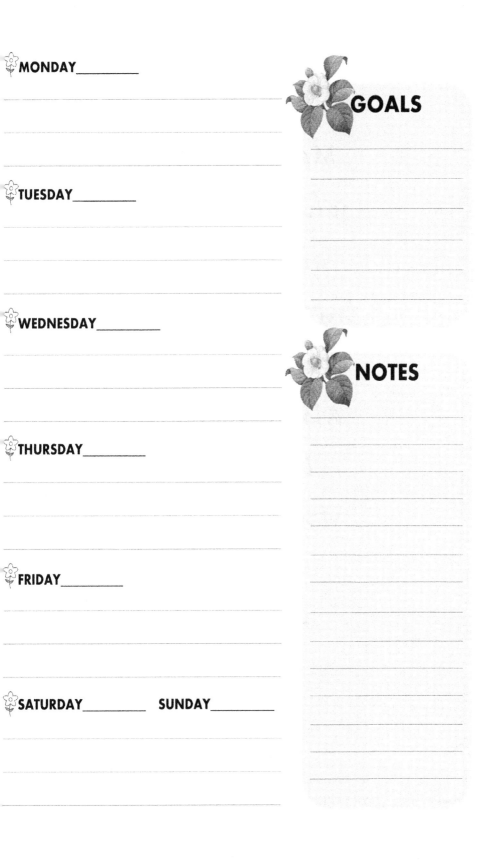

MONDAY_____

TUESDAY_____

WEDNESDAY_____

THURSDAY_____

FRIDAY_____

SATURDAY_____   **SUNDAY**_____

GOALS

NOTES

Magic happens
when you do not
give up, even
though you want
to. The universe
always falls in
love with a
stubborn heart.

-Unknown

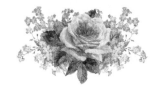

MONDAY_____

_____

_____

_____

TUESDAY_____

_____

_____

_____

WEDNESDAY_____

_____

_____

GOALS

_____

_____

_____

_____

_____

THURSDAY_____

_____

_____

NOTES

_____

_____

_____

_____

_____

FRIDAY_____

_____

_____

_____

SATURDAY_____   **SUNDAY**_____

_____

_____

_____

_____

To love someone means to see him as God intended him.

-Fyodor Dostoyevsky

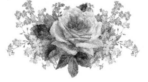

MONDAY＿＿＿＿＿

_____

_____

_____

TUESDAY＿＿＿＿＿

_____

_____

_____

WEDNESDAY＿＿＿＿＿

_____

_____

_____

THURSDAY＿＿＿＿＿

_____

_____

_____

FRIDAY＿＿＿＿＿

_____

_____

_____

SATURDAY＿＿＿＿＿   **SUNDAY**＿＿＿＿＿

_____

_____

GOALS

_____

_____

_____

_____

_____

_____

NOTES

_____

_____

_____

_____

_____

_____

_____

_____

_____

_____

_____

_____

_____

_____

_____

Beware the barrenness of a busy life.

-Socrates

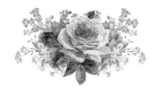

MONDAY_____

_____

_____

TUESDAY_____

_____

_____

WEDNESDAY_____

_____

_____

THURSDAY_____

_____

_____

FRIDAY_____

_____

_____

SATURDAY_____   **SUNDAY**_____

_____

_____

GOALS

_____

_____

_____

_____

_____

NOTES

_____

_____

_____

_____

_____

_____

_____

_____

_____

_____

_____

_____

_____

True knowledge
exists in
knowing that
you know
nothing.

-Socrates

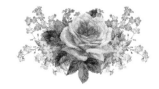

MONDAY_____

TUESDAY_____

WEDNESDAY_____

THURSDAY_____

FRIDAY_____

SATURDAY_____   **SUNDAY**_____

GOALS

NOTES

Ask and it will
be given to you;
seek and you
will find; knock
and the door will
be opened to you.

-Jesus Christ

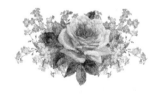

MONDAY_____

_____

_____

TUESDAY_____

_____

_____

WEDNESDAY_____

_____

_____

THURSDAY_____

_____

_____

FRIDAY_____

_____

_____

SATURDAY_____   **SUNDAY**_____

_____

_____

GOALS

_____

_____

_____

_____

_____

_____

NOTES

_____

_____

_____

_____

_____

_____

_____

_____

_____

_____

_____

_____

Not what we
have but what
we enjoy,
constitutes our
abundance.

-Epicurus

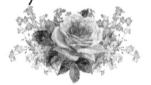

MONDAY_____

_____
_____
_____

TUESDAY_____

_____
_____
_____

WEDNESDAY_____

_____
_____

THURSDAY_____

_____
_____
_____

FRIDAY_____

_____
_____

SATURDAY_____ **SUNDAY**_____

_____
_____

GOALS

_____
_____
_____
_____
_____

NOTES

_____
_____
_____
_____
_____
_____
_____
_____
_____
_____
_____
_____
_____

Whatever you think you can do or believe you can do, begin it. Action has magic, grace and power in it.

-Johann Wolfgang von Goethe

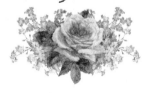

MONDAY_____

_____

_____

_____

TUESDAY_____

_____

_____

_____

WEDNESDAY_____

_____

_____

THURSDAY_____

_____

_____

_____

FRIDAY_____

_____

_____

_____

SATURDAY_____ **SUNDAY**_____

_____

_____

_____

GOALS

_____

_____

_____

_____

_____

NOTES

_____

_____

_____

_____

_____

_____

_____

_____

_____

_____

_____

_____

_____

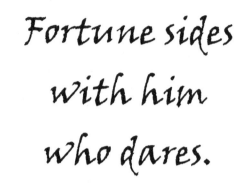

Fortune sides
with him
who dares.

-Virgil

MONDAY_____

_____

_____

GOALS

_____

TUESDAY_____

_____

_____

_____

_____

_____

WEDNESDAY_____

_____

NOTES

_____

THURSDAY_____

_____

_____

_____

_____

FRIDAY_____

_____

_____

_____

SATURDAY_____   SUNDAY_____

_____

_____

_____

From a certain
point onward
there is no longer
any turning
back. That is
the point that
must be reached.

-Franz Kafka

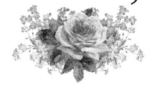

MONDAY_____

TUESDAY_____

WEDNESDAY_____

THURSDAY_____

FRIDAY_____

SATURDAY_____   **SUNDAY**_____

GOALS

NOTES

In a gentle way,
you can shake
the world.

-Mahatma
Gandhi

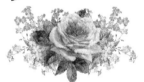

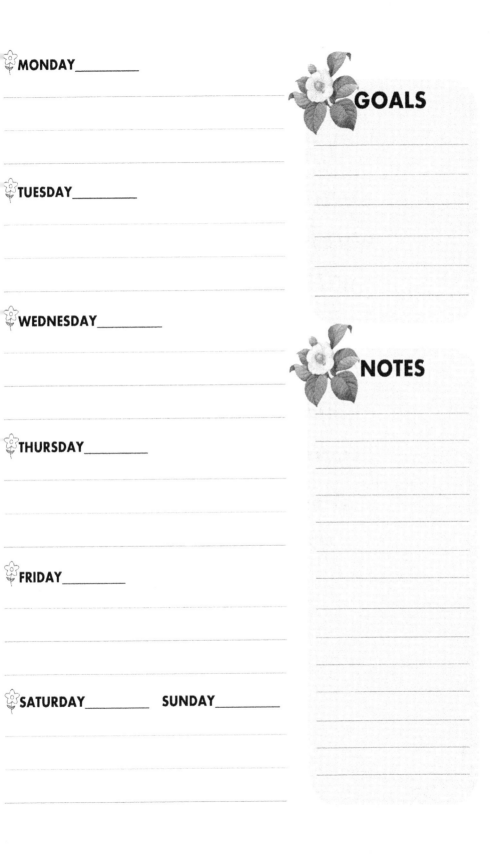

MONDAY_____

TUESDAY_____

WEDNESDAY_____

THURSDAY_____

FRIDAY_____

SATURDAY_____ **SUNDAY**_____

GOALS

NOTES

If you will know
yourselves, then you
will be known and you
will know that you
are the sons of the
living father. But if
you do not know
yourselves, then you
are in poverty and
you are poverty.

-Jesus Christ

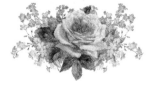

MONDAY_____

_____

_____

TUESDAY_____

_____

_____

WEDNESDAY_____

_____

THURSDAY_____

_____

_____

FRIDAY_____

_____

_____

SATURDAY_____   **SUNDAY**_____

_____

_____

GOALS

_____

_____

_____

_____

_____

NOTES

_____

_____

_____

_____

_____

_____

_____

_____

_____

_____

_____

_____

_____

_____

Of all the things
which wisdom
provides to make us
entirely happy,
much the greatest
is the possession of
friendship.

-Epicurus

MONDAY_____

_____

_____

TUESDAY_____

_____

_____

WEDNESDAY_____

_____

_____

THURSDAY_____

_____

_____

FRIDAY_____

_____

_____

SATURDAY_____   **SUNDAY**_____

GOALS

NOTES

Do not speak of
your happiness
to one less
fortunate than
yourself.

-Plutarch

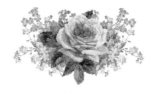

MONDAY_____

_____

_____

_____

TUESDAY_____

_____

_____

_____

WEDNESDAY_____

_____

_____

_____

THURSDAY_____

_____

_____

_____

FRIDAY_____

_____

_____

_____

SATURDAY_____   **SUNDAY**_____

_____

_____

_____

GOALS

_____

_____

_____

_____

_____

NOTES

_____

_____

_____

_____

_____

_____

_____

_____

_____

_____

_____

_____

_____

The most
powerful
weapon on earth
is the human
soul on fire.

-Marshall
Ferdinand Foch

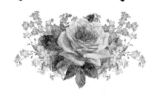

MONDAY_____

_____

_____

_____

TUESDAY_____

_____

_____

_____

WEDNESDAY_____

_____

_____

_____

THURSDAY_____

_____

_____

_____

FRIDAY_____

_____

_____

_____

SATURDAY_____   **SUNDAY**_____

_____

_____

_____

GOALS

_____

_____

_____

_____

_____

NOTES

_____

_____

_____

_____

_____

_____

_____

_____

_____

_____

_____

_____

_____

_____

_____

_____

He is richest who
is content with
the least, for
content is
the wealth
of nature.

-Socrates

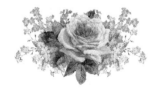

MONDAY_____

TUESDAY_____

WEDNESDAY_____

THURSDAY_____

FRIDAY_____

SATURDAY_____ **SUNDAY**_____

GOALS

NOTES

The greatest
thing in the
world is to know
how to belong
to oneself.

-Michel de
Montaigne

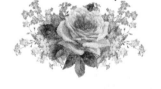

MONDAY_____

_____

_____

TUESDAY_____

_____

_____

WEDNESDAY_____

_____

_____

THURSDAY_____

_____

_____

FRIDAY_____

_____

_____

SATURDAY_____ **SUNDAY**_____

_____

_____

GOALS

_____
_____
_____
_____
_____

NOTES

_____
_____
_____
_____
_____
_____
_____
_____
_____
_____
_____
_____
_____
_____
_____
_____

Think like a
wise man but
communicate in
the language of
the people.

-W.B. Yeats

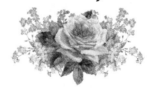

MONDAY_____

_____
_____
_____

TUESDAY_____

_____
_____
_____

WEDNESDAY_____

_____
_____

THURSDAY_____

_____
_____
_____

FRIDAY_____

_____
_____

SATURDAY_____   **SUNDAY**_____

_____
_____

GOALS

_____
_____
_____
_____
_____

NOTES

_____
_____
_____
_____
_____
_____
_____
_____
_____
_____
_____
_____
_____
_____

Love all, trust a few, do wrong to none.

-William Shakespeare

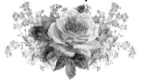

MONDAY_____

TUESDAY_____

WEDNESDAY_____

THURSDAY_____

FRIDAY_____

SATURDAY_____   SUNDAY_____

GOALS

NOTES

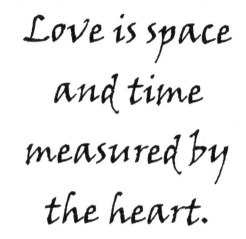

Love is space
and time
measured by
the heart.

-Marcel Proust

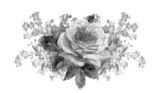

MONDAY_____

_____

_____

_____

GOALS

_____

_____

_____

TUESDAY_____

_____

_____

_____

WEDNESDAY_____

_____

_____

NOTES

_____

THURSDAY_____

_____

_____

_____

_____

FRIDAY_____

_____

_____

_____

_____

SATURDAY_____   **SUNDAY**_____

_____

_____

Blessed is he who
expects nothing,
for he shall
never be
disappointed.

-Alexander Pope

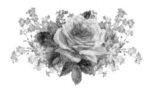

MONDAY_____

TUESDAY_____

WEDNESDAY_____

THURSDAY_____

FRIDAY_____

SATURDAY_____   SUNDAY_____

GOALS

NOTES

You have as
much laughter
as you
have faith.

-Martin Luther

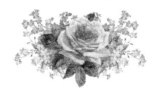

MONDAY_____

TUESDAY_____

WEDNESDAY_____

THURSDAY_____

FRIDAY_____

SATURDAY_____   **SUNDAY**_____

GOALS

NOTES

It is necessary to
have wished for
death in order to
know how good
it is to live.

-Alexandre
Dumas

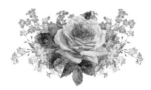

MONDAY_____

GOALS

TUESDAY_____

WEDNESDAY_____

NOTES

THURSDAY_____

FRIDAY_____

SATURDAY_____   **SUNDAY**_____

Don't bend; don't water it down; don't try to make it logical; don't edit your own soul according to the fashion. Rather, follow your most intense obsessions mercilessly.

-Franz Kafka

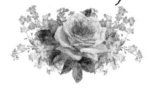

MONDAY_____

_____

_____

_____

TUESDAY_____

_____

_____

_____

WEDNESDAY_____

_____

_____

THURSDAY_____

_____

_____

_____

FRIDAY_____

_____

_____

_____

SATURDAY_____   SUNDAY_____

_____

_____

_____

GOALS

NOTES

Magic is believing
in yourself, if you
can do that,
you can make
anything happen.

-Johann Wolfgang
von Goethe

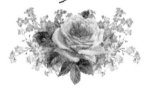

MONDAY_____

GOALS

TUESDAY_____

WEDNESDAY_____

NOTES

THURSDAY_____

FRIDAY_____

SATURDAY_____   **SUNDAY**_____

In order to
attain the
impossible, one
must attempt
the absurd.

-Miguel de
Cervantes

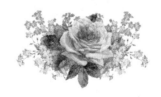

MONDAY_____

_____

_____

_____

TUESDAY_____

_____

_____

WEDNESDAY_____

_____

_____

THURSDAY_____

_____

_____

FRIDAY_____

_____

_____

SATURDAY_____   **SUNDAY**_____

_____

GOALS

_____

_____

_____

_____

_____

_____

NOTES

_____

_____

_____

_____

_____

_____

_____

_____

_____

_____

_____

_____

Diligence is
the mother of
good fortune.

-Miguel de
Cervantes

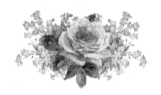

MONDAY_____

_____

_____

_____

TUESDAY_____

_____

_____

_____

WEDNESDAY_____

_____

_____

_____

THURSDAY_____

_____

_____

_____

FRIDAY_____

_____

_____

_____

SATURDAY_____ **SUNDAY**_____

_____

_____

_____

GOALS

NOTES

There is no great
genius without
a mixture
of madness.

-Aristotle

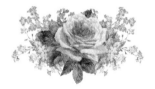

MONDAY_____

_____

_____

TUESDAY_____

_____

_____

WEDNESDAY_____

_____

_____

THURSDAY_____

_____

_____

FRIDAY_____

_____

_____

SATURDAY_____   **SUNDAY**_____

_____

GOALS

_____

_____

_____

_____

_____

NOTES

_____

_____

_____

_____

_____

_____

_____

_____

_____

_____

_____

_____

_____

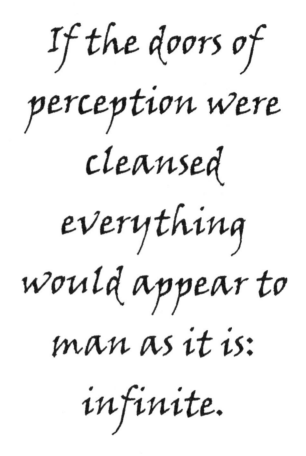

If the doors of
perception were
cleansed
everything
would appear to
man as it is:
infinite.

-William Blake

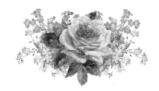

MONDAY_____

GOALS

TUESDAY_____

WEDNESDAY_____

NOTES

THURSDAY_____

FRIDAY_____

SATURDAY_____ **SUNDAY**_____

That which
does not kill
us makes us
stronger.

-Friedrich
Nietzsche

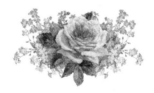

MONDAY_____

_____

_____

_____

TUESDAY_____

_____

_____

_____

WEDNESDAY_____

_____

_____

_____

THURSDAY_____

_____

_____

_____

FRIDAY_____

_____

_____

_____

SATURDAY_____   **SUNDAY**_____

_____

_____

GOALS

_____

_____

_____

_____

_____

NOTES

_____

_____

_____

_____

_____

_____

_____

_____

_____

_____

_____

_____

_____

Made in the USA
Las Vegas, NV
11 March 2022

45415122R00059